NEONATAL NURSING:
SCOPE AND STANDARDS
OF PRACTICE

AMERICAN NURSES
ASSOCIATION

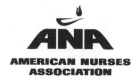

Washington, D.C.
2004

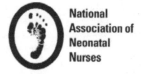

National
Association of
Neonatal
Nurses

Library of Congress Cataloging-in-Publication data

Neonatal nursing : scope and standards of practice.
   p. ; cm.
Includes bibliographical references and index.
ISBN 1-55810-222-1
1. Infants (Newborn)--Diseases--Nursing--Standards.
[DNLM: 1. Neonatal Nursing--standards. WY 157.3 N4388 2004]
I. American Nurses Association. II. National Association of Neonatal Nurses.

RJ253.N443 2004
618.92'00231--dc22
                          2004011997

RJ253
.N443
2004
o 55494894

The American Nurses Association (ANA) is a national professional association. This ANA publication—*Neonatal Nursing: Scope and Standards of Practice*—reflects the thinking of the nursing profession on various issues and should be reviewed in conjunction with state board of nursing policies and practices. State law, rules, and regulations govern the practice of nursing, while *Neonatal Nursing: Scope and Standards of Practice* guides nurses in the application of their professional skills and responsibilities.

Published by nursesbooks.org
The Publishing Program of ANA

American Nurses Association
600 Maryland Avenue, SW • Suite 100 West • Washington, DC 20024
1-800-274-4ANA • http://www.nursingworld.org/

ISBN 1-55810-222-1
04SSVN   2M   05/04

ACKNOWLEDGEMENTS

This document was developed by the National Association of Neonatal Nurses (NANN) Scope and Standards Practice Task Force. The members of the task force gratefully acknowledge the work of the previous task forces that initiated the original documents on neonatal nursing practice. Carole Kenner, DNS RNC FAAN, especially is thanked for her review of the early drafts of this document.

The early versions of *Neonatal Nursing: Scope and Standards of Practice* were modified based on the thoughtful comments and editing suggestions of volunteer reviewers and from the pre-publication review by the NANN Board of Directors.

NANN Scope and Standards Task Force
Susan Stang, MSN, RNC, APN, Task Force Chair
Leda Afuang, MSN, RNC, LNC
Wendy Bedran, BSN, RN
Janet Geyer, MSN, RN, ARNP
Karen Goldschmidt, BSN, RNC
Cheryl King, MSN, CCRN

NANN Staff Liaisons
Brandon Dybala
Louise S. Miller, MA

NANN Board of Directors, 2003–2004
Catherine Witt, MS, RNC, NNP, President
Robin Bissinger, MSN, RNC, NNP, President-Elect
Peggy Gordin, MS, RNC, NNP, FAAN, Secretary
Suzanne Staebler, MSN, RNC, NNP, Treasurer
Margaret Conway-Orgel, MSN, RNC, NNP, Past President
Priscilla Frappier, MPH, MS, RNC, NNP, Director at Large
Karin Gracey, MSN, RNC, CNNP, Director at Large
Karen Kopischke, MS, RNC, NNP, Director at Large
Lori Sellers, MSN, RN, Director at Large
Cynthia Weiss, RNC, Director at Large
Linda Juretschke, MSN RNC NNP, Special Interest Group (SIG) Director at Large

American Nurses Association (ANA) Staff
Carol J. Bickford, PhD, RN,BC, Content Editor
Yvonne Humes, MSA
Winifred Carson-Smith, JD

CONTENTS

INTRODUCTION

Neonatal nursing, as a specialty, has developed significantly during the past 40 years. Specialty care for the sick or premature infant began with the invention of the incubator in 1878 and its subsequent display with infants at world expositions and fairs until the 1940s. In 1923 the first hospital center for premature infants in the United States was established, and in 1950 the first federal grant funding the Premature Institute program to train hospitals in caring for this special group of newborns was provided. These developments led to the expanded role of nurses into specialized nursing care for the neonate in the early 1960s and the country's first neonatal intensive care unit (NICU).

Advances in technology and health care led to regionalization in most large teaching hospitals and the development of high-tech neonatal care during the 1970s. The American College of Obstetricians and Gynecologists added validity to the specialty with the publication of standards of care for neonates. In turn, neonatal nurses developed their skills and advanced their roles in infant care as nurse clinicians, practitioners, clinical specialists, and educators.

As these well-trained nurses increased in number, they developed associations to further their knowledge and expertise. Developing from the Neonatal Nurses of Northern California, the Neonatal Nurses Association, and the Neonatal Nurse Clinicians Practitioners & Specialists, in 1984 the National Association of Neonatal Nurses (NANN) was born. Since its inception, NANN has provided the opportunity to specialize neonatal nursing further by consolidating the voice of its members and creating support and unity in this unique nursing field.

To help the profession and the public better understand the practice of neonatal nursing and thereby value today's neonatal nurses, the National Association of Neonatal Nurses convened the Scope and Standards of Practice Task Force to examine historical documents, references, and resources and then create the specialty's scope and standards of practice. This work identified key assumptions that guided further thinking and proved integral to the development of the scope of practice statement. (These assumptions are listed on page ix). The scope of practice statement provides the answers to the *who, what, where, when, why,* and *how* questions about the neonatal nursing specialty.

The standards for neonatal nursing practice are generic statements that define the responsibilities and accountability to the profession and the public of all registered nurses who care for high-risk neonates and their families.

These standards reflect the values and priorities of the profession of nursing as they relate to the specialty of neonatal nursing and provide directives and a measurement framework for minimal levels of care that are common to the registered nurse in the neonatal nursing field.

The specialty scope and standards of practice must be considered in relation to the definition of nursing and other content in *Nursing's Social Policy Statement, 2nd Edition* (2003) and *Code of Ethics for Nurses with Interpretive Statements* (2001). As well, it must be reviewed and revised on a regular basis to reflect changes in health care and the nursing profession. In 2004, *Neonatal Nursing: Scope and Standards of Practice* completed the American Nurses Association's established review and recognition process for specialty nursing scope and standards of practice.

Considered together, *standards of practice* and *standards of professional performance* (ANA, 2004) encompass minimally acceptable levels of nursing care and nursing performance. The *standards of practice* include the steps in the nursing process: assessment, diagnosis, planning, implementation, and evaluation. In today's climate of cost containment and evidence-based practice, it must also include outcomes of care. The *standards of professional performance* include quality of care, performance appraisal, education, collegiality, ethics, collaboration, research, resource utilization, and leadership (ANA, 2004, p. 3). The professional nurse is expected to be competent and accountable in these areas of nursing practice.

Underlying Assumptions

The following assumptions were made in the development of *Neonatal Nursing: Scope and Standards of Practice*:

1. The standards focus primarily on the process of providing nursing care to newborns/infants and their families.
2. The healthcare facility will provide a sufficient number of qualified registered nurses to deliver safe and effective neonatal nursing care.
3. Nursing care is individualized to meet the unique needs of each newborn/infant and family.
4. The nurse considers and respects the family's goals and preferences when developing and implementing a plan of care.
5. The nurse respects the cultural aspects of newborn/infant and family care.
6. The nurse respects the rights of the newborn/infant and family and manages information accordingly.
7. The nurse provides information to the family so informed decisions can be made regarding the care of the newborn/infant and family.
8. The nurse functions within the Nurse Practice Acts of the state and the established policies and procedures as described by the healthcare institution in which the nurse is practicing.
9. Nursing care is administered considering the rights of the patient and family, as outlined by the institution. Such care is given with regard for the family's spiritual and cultural values, in a manner that is ethically relevant, based on scientific knowledge, and within the confines of the legal system.
10. The nurse works in coordination with other healthcare providers to render care to the newborn/infant and family.
11. The nurse is expected to continue and maintain education within the neonatal specialty.
12. The nurse strives to provide a high quality of care while utilizing available resources.
13. The nurse promotes collegiality and collaboration in an effort to provide holistic care.
14. The nurse recognizes ethical dilemmas and use appropriate resources to work through these situations.
16. The nurse strives to ensure use of evidence-based care when possible and identify the need for research in areas lacking evidence to support practice.

Standards of Neonatal Nursing Practice: Standards of Practice

STANDARD 1. ASSESSMENT
The neonatal nurse collects comprehensive data on the healthcare needs of the infant and family.

STANDARD 2. DIAGNOSIS
The neonatal nurse formulates diagnoses based on analysis and synthesis of assessment data.

STANDARD 3. OUTCOME IDENTIFICATION
The neonatal nurse identifies expected individualized outcomes of care based on the needs of the infant and family.

STANDARD 4. PLANNING
The neonatal nurse develops a plan of care that prescribes interventions to attain expected outcomes.

STANDARD 5. IMPLEMENTATION
The neonatal nurse implements the plan of care.

STANDARD 5A: COORDINATION OF CARE
The neonatal nurse coordinates care delivery.

STANDARD 5B: HEALTH TEACHING AND HEALTH PROMOTION
The neonatal nurse employs strategies to promote health and a safe environment.

STANDARD 5C: CONSULTATION
The advanced practice registered nurse provides consultation to influence the identified plan, enhance the abilities of others, and effect change.

STANDARD 5D: PRESCRIPTIVE AUTHORITY AND TREATMENT
The advanced practice registered nurse uses prescriptive authority, procedures, referrals, treatments, and therapies in accordance with state and federal laws and regulations.

STANDARD 6. EVALUATION
The neonatal nurse evaluates the progress of the infant and family toward the attainment of established, expected outcomes.

STANDARDS OF
NEONATAL NURSING PRACTICE:
STANDARDS OF PROFESSIONAL PERFORMANCE

STANDARD 7. QUALITY OF PRACTICE
The neonatal nurse systematically evaluates the quality and effectiveness of nursing practice.

STANDARD 8. EDUCATION
The neonatal nurse acquires and maintains current knowledge and competency in nursing practice.

STANDARD 9. PROFESSIONAL PRACTICE EVALUATION
The neonatal nurse evaluates one's own nursing practice in relation to professional practice standards and guidelines, relevant statutes, rules, and regulations.

STANDARD 10. COLLEGIALITY
The neonatal nurse interacts with, and contributes to the professional development of, peers, other healthcare providers, and team members as colleagues.

STANDARD 11. COLLABORATION
The neonatal nurse collaborates with the family or caregiver and others in the conduct of nursing practice.

STANDARD 12. ETHICS
The neonatal nurse's decisions and actions on behalf of infants and their families or caregivers in all areas of practice are determined in an ethical manner.

STANDARD 13. RESEARCH
The neonatal nurse integrates research findings into practice.

STANDARD 14. RESOURCE UTILIZATION
The neonatal nurse considers factors related to safety, effectiveness, cost, and impact on practice in the planning and delivering of nursing services.

STANDARD 15. LEADERSHIP
The neonatal nurse provides leadership in the professional practice setting and the profession.

NEONATAL NURSING SCOPE OF PRACTICE

Neonatal nursing is the specialized care of the neonate, infant, and family from birth and hospitalization to discharge and follow-up care. Traditionally, this highly specialized nursing practice encompasses the care of infants born preterm, term, or ill from complications detected pre- or postnatally. Currently, the specialty has evolved to encompass care of the infant up to one year of age with problems that stem from complications of prematurity or other newborn illness. The neonatal nurse recognizes and respects each infant as a unique, individual human being, with the right to a pain-free, developmentally supportive care environment. The nurse assists the family's adaptation to a new, highly technical environment, while encouraging attachment to and bonding with their newborn. The neonatal nurse recognizes the family's attachment to the newborn as crucial for the infant's physical, psychological, and emotional wellbeing, growth, and development. The goal of the neonatal nurse is to empower the family through education, practice, and competence in caring for their newborn.

Practice Characteristics

Neonatal nurses understand complex newborn disease processes and acquire the expertise needed to utilize state-of-the-art technology to care for neonates and infants. The neonatal nurse has the ability to assess and manage care of the newborn infant and is able to respond appropriately to serious or life-threatening conditions. The neonatal nurse makes skilled, knowledgeable assessments of the infant, anticipates illness, and whenever possible prevents the occurrence of illness and injury or minimizes its effect. In caring for newborn infants, the neonatal nurse recognizes the importance of holistic care and supports the family's adaptive coping. Specific phenomena that form the framework for neonatal nursing practice include the following:

- *Communication:* Continual direct observation of the infant unable to communicate verbally is vital. The neonatal nurse detects subtle changes in the infant's physiological status and communicates these changes to the physician, advanced practice nurse, and family. The neonatal nurse works in collaboration with the healthcare team, including physicians, advanced practice nurses, case managers, laboratory technicians, occupational, physical, and respiratory therapists, nutritionists, social workers, and childlife specialists, to provide optimal care for the fragile newborn and family.

- *Culturally Sensitive Care:* The neonatal nurse provides culturally sensitive care to the infant and family by understanding the family's unique cultural needs while caring for the newborn. Family-centered, culturally appropriate care can eliminate potential barriers to health care for the family and is essential for the infant's wellbeing (NANN, 1999b).

- *Developmental Care:* The neonatal nurse provides care for medically fragile infants while supporting their development, thereby enhancing the infant's growth and neurodevelopmental potential.

- *Health Promotion:* In planning and providing care, the neonatal nurse considers all aspects of the infant's health, including preventive health care. The neonatal nurse closely assesses the infant's physiological status, develops a specialized plan of care, and evaluates the infant's response. The neonatal nurse devises, coordinates, and executes an individualized plan of care for the newborn, revising plans as needed, and continually evaluates responses from the infant and family.

- *Environment:* The neonatal nurse recognizes the significant effects of the environment on the health of the newborn. The neonatal nurse identifies and treats pain and prevents suffering through management of the infant's discomfort with both independent nursing interventions and medications. The nurse strives to eliminate or minimize negative iatrogenic effects for the infant and to provide a nurturing environment; coordinates care to provide the infant with uninterrupted sleep periods; monitors the infant's temperature, comfort level, and nutritional needs; monitors the ambient lighting and noise level in the unit; and provides protection from infection. The neonatal nurse promotes positive family–infant interaction through holding, kangaroo care, breast or bottle feeding, and involvement in the infant's daily-care needs.

- *Discharge Planning:* The neonatal nurse plays an important role in preparing the family or caregivers for discharge of sick, medically fragile, or recovering term or preterm infants. The neonatal nurse must be knowledgeable of current, evidence-based discharge practices, and community resources to ease transition of infant and family into the home environment.

- *Ethical Decision-Making:* In practice, the neonatal nurse is challenged with ethical decisions daily. The nurse works in conjunction with physicians, advanced practice nurses, and family to provide care that is determined to be in the best interest of the child. The neonatal nurse acknowledges the parents' role as spokespersons for the infant. The neonatal nurse acts as infant advocate, providing the family with detailed information to enable fact-based decision-making and informed consent. The neonatal nurse identifies potential ethical conflicts and coordinates interdisciplinary forums for discussion and resolution.

Neonatal Nursing: Scope and Standards of Practice

- *Family-Focused Care:* Neonatal nurses recognize the family as an integral part of the healthcare team, as well as the importance of the family's role in enhancing the developmental outcome of the infant. The neonatal nurse assists the family in caring for the newborn, whether that means teaching basic newborn care or teaching a family how to care for their medically fragile infant in the home. The nurse recognizes the infant's need of a family competent in physical care, as well as in interpreting behavioral cues.

- *Spiritual Care:* The neonatal nurse plays an integral role in helping families cope with hope and joy, as well as grief and loss. Extended hospitalization of the newborn is recognized as a family crisis. The neonatal nurse recognizes that grieving is individual and occurs in stages. The neonatal nurse learns and respects religious and spiritual family practices, while conveying acceptance, openness, and availability. The neonatal nurse assists the families and the infant at the end of life however possible.

- *Quality Assurance and Research:* The neonatal nurse utilizes research-based nursing practice to provide quality nursing care to the newborn. The nurse participates in identifying potential research studies to benefit the newborn and the practice of neonatal nursing care.

Practice Environment, Education, Certification, and Roles

The neonatal nurse provides health care to the infant in a variety of settings, including the delivery room, newborn nursery, and the subacute care, acute care, chronic care, transport, home care, and infant follow-up clinics. In the hospital setting, neonatal units are regionalized to provide care for specified infant-acuity levels. These units are typically described by the level of care they provide. The neonatal nurse has the opportunity to practice in environments with infants of varying degrees of acuity:

- *Delivery Room:* The neonatal nurse is responsible for attending the birth of every neonate deemed to be at high risk. Knowledge of common causes of infant distress at birth requiring neonatal resuscitation is essential. A nurse trained in neonatal resuscitation is responsible for rapid and accurate evaluation of the newborn at delivery.

- *Level I:* At this level of care, the nurse directly observes the neonate during the stabilization period after birth. The nurse monitors the infant's adaptation to extrauterine life and then ideally assists transition of the newborn to rooming in with the mother. The neonatal nurse can also practice in a newborn nursery taking care of healthy newborns. This level of care is an essential part of mother–infant care.

- *Level II:* In the Level II setting, often referred to as special care or transitional care, the neonatal nurse takes on a greater responsibility for monitoring the premature newborn or the newborn who is having difficulty in adapting to extrauterine life. The neonatal nurse at this level cares for premature or term newborns who are ill or injured from complications at birth. The neonatal nurse provides the newborn with frequent observation and monitoring. The infants in this unit may require respiratory support, supplemental oxygen, intravenous therapy, specialized feeding, or time to mature prior to discharge. The nurse provides the family with discharge instruction and arranges for follow-up support when the infant is discharged to home.

- *Level III:* In the Level III unit (NICU), the neonatal nurse is challenged by treating the acutely ill newborn during a critical period. Expert care and knowledge are required in this highly technical and challenging environment. In the Level III neonatal unit, the nurse provides direct care for the premature or term infant who requires complex care. The neonatal nurse in this unit cares for the infant requiring intensive life-support techniques, such as mechanical ventilation, nitric oxide therapy, and high-frequency ventilation. Select Level III intensive care units have the added capability to care for an infant requiring extracorporeal membrane oxygenation (ECMO). The nurse in these units also cares for the chronically technology-dependent infant. The nurse teaches the family how to care for the child in the home setting or aids in the transition to a rehabilitation center (Bagwell et al, 2003).

- *Transport:* The neonatal nurse may be responsible for transporting an infant via ground or air. For those infants born acutely ill in a location without the necessary resources, the neonatal nurse assists the physician or advanced practice nurse in the transport to a tertiary care center (NANN, 1999c). The neonatal transport nurse is responsible for assessment, stabilization, and continuous high-level care during the transfer to the tertiary care center. The neonatal nurse may also be responsible for transporting the stable newborn back to the referring institution or a rehabilitation center.

The care of the neonatal patient is guided by the neonatal nursing standards of practice. At all care levels the neonatal nurse recognizes the importance of their role as an infant and family advocate. Training to assess minute changes in the infant's health and to observe unspoken cues and physiological changes define this nursing practice. The neonatal nurse evaluates outcomes of the infant's care and revises the plan as necessary to promote wellness. Sick newborns require the attention of specialized, expert neonatal nurses at all care levels.

Graduation from an accredited nursing program and registered nursing licensure are required for entry into the field of neonatal nursing. An appropriate orientation program supports the registered nurse in initial practice. This program provides the nurse new to the field with the opportunity to work with an experienced neonatal nurse. The professional neonatal nurse is encouraged to meet their learning needs through professional development experiences, such as continuing education opportunities, conferences in neonatal care, and involvement in a professional nursing organization pertinent to practice.

Advanced practice neonatal nursing (APN) requires additional formal education at the master's degree level. The APN is an expert practitioner in the role of either nurse practitioner or clinical nurse specialist, who collaborates with neonatologists, pediatricians, and the infant's family (NANN, 1999a). The neonatal nurse practitioner (NNP) is a master's-prepared nurse who is responsible for managing a case load of infants, in collaboration with the neonatologist. The NNP typically is responsible for medical and nursing management of their patients, but also may be responsible for educating staff and developing standards of care. The neonatal clinical nurse specialist (NCNS), another master's-prepared neonatal nurse, is responsible for fostering continuous quality improvement in neonatal nursing care. The NCNS develops and educates staff, models expert nursing practice, and applies and promotes evidence-based nursing practice. Doctorate-prepared neonatal nurses may focus on conducting research to test caregiving practices and develop theory, while some are clinically focused. Both master's- and doctorate-prepared advanced practice neonatal nurses can teach neonatal nursing in the college or hospital setting (Harrigan et al, 2003).

Professionalism in neonatal nursing is demonstrated by assuming accountability for maintaining excellence in practice through self-motivated ventures as well as collaborative efforts with other nursing colleagues, organizations, and professional associations. Participation in the specialty's certification process further demonstrates the nurse's expertise in neonatal nursing. Nurses who have worked in neonatal nursing for a minimum of 2 years may choose to test their proficiency in neonatal nursing to become certified in either low-risk or high-risk neonatal nursing. Certification may be retained through continuing education or retesting.

Beyond the clinical environment and the provision of direct patient care, the neonatal nurse may practice in a variety of roles: clinical nurse specialist, educator, researcher, consultant, and clinical expert. Basic nursing roles include staff nurse, primary nurse, delivery room nurse, neonatal transport nurse, special care nurse, or transitional nursery nurse with varying degrees of advancement. Advanced-practice titles include clinical nurse specialist or nurse practitioner.

Future Considerations

As technology advances, it may become possible to care for infants previously considered nonviable. The neonatal nurse's role will change as new technology and treatments are devised. Advances in infertility treatment continue to increase the need for neonatal nurses as the numbers of multiple births and high-risk deliveries increase.

Today, neonates are being discharged earlier than ever. There is a growing need for neonatal nurses to care for the newborn in the home. The nurse in this capacity will provide follow-up visits as well as technically advanced care for infants in the home. This trend requires well-developed care plans and communication between the NICU team and the home-care agency (Harrigan et al, 2003).

DNA testing and advances in gene therapy may have future implications for neonatal nurses. These advances may lead the way to preventing adverse genetic traits from being passed to future generations, thus preventing diseases such as Huntington's, Thalassaemia, Cystic Fibrosis, and Sickle Cell Disease. Another area of genetic research, Pharmacogenomics, (combining genetics and pharmaceuticals) may enable medications to be adapted to an individual's genetic makeup, yielding more targeted drugs with fewer side effects, and replacing weight- and age-based dosing (Human Genome Project, 2004).

Fetal surgery has implications for this profession, merging the roles of the delivery room nurse, surgical nurse, and neonatal nurse. This type of surgery has the potential for creating new patient populations.

Ethical decision-making will continue to be an important part of the nurse's daily work, possibly becoming increasingly complex. It is important that neonatal nurses are nurtured and supported in this stressful environment. Recruitment and retention of neonatal nursing staff and support of new graduates entering the profession are crucial for the advancement and survival of the profession.

Through research, the neonatal nurse should strive to develop evidence-based practice guidelines. Much of the research in neonatology at present is physician-driven. The neonatal nurse has the opportunity to make changes in practice through scientifically grounded research studies. This will enable the neonatal nursing profession to grow and gain further professional credibility (Stevens, 2003).

Due to all of the influences on preterm births, there will be a growing need for neonatal nurses in the future. There is a shortage of acute-care neonatal nurses, which is projected to continue into the next decade. Many health insurance plans are now providing reimbursement for the services of the APN and NNP in managing the low-risk and intermediate nursery in collaboration with physicians, because their services have proven to be advantageous and cost-effective.

STANDARDS OF NEONATAL NURSING PRACTICE
STANDARDS OF PRACTICE FOR NEONATAL NURSING

STANDARD 1. ASSESSMENT

The neonatal nurse collects comprehensive data on the healthcare needs of the infant and family.

Measurement Criteria:

The neonatal nurse:

1. Determines the priority of data collection by the infant's and family's immediate condition and needs.

2. Collects data including antenatal and perinatal information, pertinent sociocultural data, physical assessment data, laboratory data analyses, and diagnostic testing.

3. Collects pertinent data using appropriate assessment techniques.

4. Utilizes data sources including family members, significant others, and other healthcare providers. Reassessment should be completed within a reasonable time, to ensure that the needs of the infant and family continue to be met.

5. Employs a data collection process that is systematic, ongoing, and relevant to the changing healthcare needs of the infant and the learning needs of the family.

6. Collects relevant data, systematically documented in a retrievable form.

7. Analyzes data to produce information about the infant's needs for treatment and services, to identify the need for additional data, and to identify patterns and variances.

8. Collects relevant data regarding the continued needs of the infant and family during follow-up visits and convalescent periods.

9. Assesses the infant for the presence of pain, then treats and reassesses in accordance with the institution's process.

Additional Measurement Criteria for the Advanced Practice Registered Nurse:

The advanced practice registered nurse initiates and interprets diagnostic tests and procedures relevant to the infant's current status.

9

STANDARD 2. DIAGNOSIS

The neonatal nurse formulates diagnoses based on analysis and synthesis of assessment data.

Measurement Criteria:

The neonatal nurse:

1. Derives diagnoses using assessment data that reflect the infant's current clinical condition.

2. Refines and revises diagnoses regularly, based on data subsequently collected.

3. Validates diagnoses with the infant's family and other healthcare providers when possible.

4. Derives diagnoses encompassing:

    • the infant's identified or potential physiological and developmental problems,

    • the infant's integration into the family during the period of hospitalization and after discharge,

    • the support and educational needs of the family, and

    • any present or potential environmental problems.

5. Documents diagnoses in a manner that facilitates the determination of expected outcomes and the plan of care.

Additional Measurement Criteria for the Advanced Practice Registered Nurse:

The advanced practice registered nurse:

• Systematically compares and contrasts clinical findings with normal and abnormal variations and developmental events in formulating a differential diagnosis.

• Utilizes complex data and information obtained during review of history, interview, examination, and diagnostic procedures in identifying diagnoses.

• Assists staff in developing and maintaining competency in the diagnostic process.

STANDARD 3. OUTCOME IDENTIFICATION

The neonatal nurse identifies expected individualized outcomes of care based on the needs of the infant and family.

Measurement Criteria:

The neonatal nurse:

1. Derives outcomes from the assessment and relevant nursing diagnoses.

2. Identifies outcomes consistent with current scientific evidence.

3. Mutually formulates outcomes with input from other healthcare providers and the family whenever possible.

4. Ensures that outcomes are culturally appropriate and realistic in relation to the infant and the family's present and potential capabilities.

5. Derives outcomes that are attainable in relation to the resources available to the infant and the family.

6. Develops a realistic time frame for attainment of objectives.

7. Identifies outcomes that provide direction for continuity of care.

8. Derives outcomes that provide a basis for evaluating and monitoring care.

Additional Measurement Criteria for the Advanced Practice Registered Nurse:

The advanced practice registered nurse:

- Identifies expected outcomes that incorporate scientific evidence and are achievable through implementation of evidence-based practices.

- Identifies expected outcomes that incorporate cost and clinical effectiveness, family or caregiver satisfaction, and continuity and consistency among providers.

- Supports the use of clinical guidelines linked to positive infant outcomes.

STANDARD 4. PLANNING

The neonatal nurse develops a plan of care that prescribes interventions to attain expected outcomes.

Measurement Criteria:

The neonatal nurse:

1. Develops a plan that is individualized to the infant and family and is culturally, environmentally, and educationally sensitive and age-appropriate.

2. Develops the plan with the family and other healthcare providers whenever appropriate.

3. Ensures that the plan reflects current neonatal nursing practice.

4. Organizes, integrates, and plans care with consideration for the infant's stage of development.

5. Develops a plan that incorporates the family in caregiving based on the infant's condition and the family's ability to participate.

6. Ensures that the plan is systematically documented and easily retrievable.

7. Provides for continuity of care within the plan.

8. Ensures that the plan is a dynamic process that addresses the needs of the infant. It must be reevaluated within a reasonable time to ensure that the needs of the infant continue to be met.

9. Establishes the plan priorities for care with the family and other healthcare providers.

10. Integrates into the plan current trends and research affecting care in the planning process.

Additional Measurement Criteria for the Advanced Practice Registered Nurse:

The advanced practice registered nurse:

• Identifies assessment, diagnostic strategies and therapeutic interventions within the plan that reflect current evidence, including data, research, literature, and expert clinical knowledge.

• Selects or designs strategies to meet the multifaceted needs of special-care infants and their families or caregivers.

• Includes the synthesis of family or caregiver values and beliefs regarding nursing and medical therapies within the plan.

STANDARD 5. IMPLEMENTATION

The neonatal nurse implements the plan of care.

Measurement Criteria:

The neonatal nurse:

1. Ensures that implementation of care is systematic and ongoing.

2. Utilizes interventions that are consistent with the established plan of care.

3. Organizes interventions to provide an environment that supports the infant's physical and developmental wellbeing.

4. Implements interventions in a manner that promotes family involvement and acquisition of progressive caregiving skills.

5. Implements interventions in a safe, timely, and appropriate manner.

6. Documents interventions in a retrievable form.

7. Individualizes interventions based on the specific needs of the infant and family.

Additional Measurement Criteria for the Advanced Practice Registered Nurse:

The advanced practice registered nurse:

• Facilitates utilization of systems and community resources to implement the plan.

• Supports collaboration with nursing colleagues and other disciplines to implement the plan.

• Incorporates new knowledge and strategies to initiate change in nursing care practices if desired outcomes are not achieved.

STANDARD 5A: COORDINATION OF CARE

The neonatal nurse coordinates care delivery.

Measurement Criteria:

The neonatal nurse:

1. Coordinates implementation of the plan.

2. Documents the coordination of the care.

Additional Measurement Criteria for the Advanced Practice Registered Nurse:

The advanced practice registered nurse:

- Provides leadership in the coordination of multidisciplinary health care for integrated delivery of infant care services.

- Synthesizes data and information to prescribe necessary system and community support measures, including environmental modifications.

- Coordinates system and community resources that enhance delivery of care across continuums.

STANDARD 5B: HEALTH TEACHING AND HEALTH PROMOTION

The neonatal nurse employs strategies to promote health and a safe environment.

Measurement Criteria:

The neonatal nurse:

1. Provides family or caregiver teaching that addresses such topics as healthy lifestyles, risk-reducing behaviors, developmental needs, and normal/specific infant care and safety.

2. Uses health promotion and health teaching methods appropriate to the situation and the family or caregiver's developmental level, learning needs, readiness, ability to learn, language preference, and culture.

3. Seeks opportunities for feedback and evaluation of the effectiveness of the strategies used.

Additional Measurement Criteria for the Advanced Practice Registered Nurse:

The advanced practice registered nurse:

• Synthesizes empirical evidence on risk behaviors, learning theories, behavioral change theories, motivational theories, epidemiology, and other related theories and frameworks when designing health information and family or caregiver education.

• Designs health information and family or caregiver education appropriate to the family or caregiver's developmental level, learning needs, readiness to learn, and cultural values and beliefs.

• Evaluates health information resources, such as the Internet, within the area of practice for accuracy, readability, and comprehensibility to help the family or caregiver access quality health information.

STANDARD 5C: CONSULTATION

The advanced practice registered nurse provides consultation to influence the identified plan, enhance the abilities of others, and effect change.

Additional Measurement Criteria for the Advanced Practice Registered Nurse:

The advanced practice registered nurse:

- Synthesizes clinical data, theoretical frameworks, and evidence when providing consultation.

- Facilitates the effectiveness of a consultation by involving the family or caregiver in decision-making and negotiating role responsibilities.

- Communicates consultation recommendations that facilitate change.

STANDARD 5D: PRESCRIPTIVE AUTHORITY AND TREATMENT

The advanced practice registered nurse uses prescriptive authority, procedures, referrals, treatments, and therapies in accordance with state and federal laws and regulations.

Additional Measurement Criteria for the Advanced Practice Registered Nurse:

The advanced practice registered nurse:

- Prescribes evidence-based treatments, therapies, and procedures considering the infant's comprehensive healthcare needs.

- Prescribes pharmacologic agents based on a current knowledge of pharmacology and physiology.

- Prescribes specific pharmacological agents or treatments based on clinical indicators, the infant's status and needs, and the results of diagnostic and laboratory tests.

- Evaluates therapeutic and potential adverse effects of pharmacological and non-pharmacological treatments.

- Provides the family or caregiver with information about intended effects and potential adverse effects of proposed prescriptive therapies.

- Provides information about costs, alternative treatments, and procedures, as appropriate.

STANDARD 6. EVALUATION

The neonatal nurse evaluates the progress of the infant and family toward the attainment of established, expected outcomes.

Measurement Criteria:

The neonatal nurse:

1. Evaluates care in a systematic, ongoing, and criterion-based manner.

2. Evaluates interventions in relation to desired, expected outcomes, and alters them when warranted.

3. Evaluates interventions based on the infant's physiological and behavioral responses, and alters them when warranted.

4. Uses ongoing assessment data to revise diagnoses, outcomes, and the plan of care as needed.

5. Systematically documents revisions in the infant's plan of care and reports to appropriate members of the healthcare team.

6. Involves the infant's family or caregivers and other healthcare providers in the evaluation process when appropriate.

7. Documents the infant's and family or caregiver's responses to interventions in a retrievable form.

Additional Measurement Criteria for the Advanced Practice Registered Nurse:

The advanced practice registered nurse:

•   Evaluates the accuracy of the diagnosis and effectiveness of the interventions in relationship to the infant's and the family's or caregiver's attainment of expected outcomes.

•   Synthesizes the results of the evaluation analyses to determine the impact of the plan on the affected infants, families, groups, communities, and institutions.

•   Uses the results of the evaluation analyses to make or recommend process or structural changes including policy, procedure or protocol documentation, as appropriate.

Standards of Professional Performance for Neonatal Nursing

The neonatal nurse systematically evaluates the quality and effectiveness of nursing practice.

Measurement Criteria:

The neonatal nurse:

1. Participates in activities to assess the quality of care that are appropriate to the nurse's education and position. These activities may include the following:

    • Identification of aspects of care that affect quality.

    • Analysis of quality data to identify opportunities for improvement of care.

    • Development of policies, procedures, and practice guidelines reflective of quality of care.

    • Identification of indicators used to monitor quality and affect neonatal care.

    • Ongoing data collection for monitoring the quality and effectiveness of nursing care.

    • Articulation of recommendations for quality improvement of nursing practice or patient outcomes.

    • Participation in interdisciplinary teams to implement activities and evaluate clinical practice or health issues.

2. Uses continuous quality-improvement activities to initiate changes in nursing practice.

3. Uses quality-improvement data to initiate healthcare delivery system changes, as needed.

4. Works in collaboration with the healthcare team to use scientific research to provide evidence-based practice.

Continued ▶

Additional Measurement Criteria for the Advanced Practice Registered Nurse:

The advanced practice registered nurse:

- Obtains and maintains professional certification in neonatal nursing.
- Designs quality improvement initiatives.
- Implements initiatives to evaluate the need for change.
- Evaluates the practice environment and quality of nursing care rendered in relation to existing evidence, identifying opportunities for research.

Standard 8. Education

The neonatal nurse acquires and maintains current knowledge and competency in nursing practice.

Measurement Criteria:

The neonatal nurse:

1. Participates in ongoing educational activities related to clinical and theoretical knowledge and professional issues.
2. Seeks experiences that reflect current clinical practice to maintain current clinical skills and competence.
3. Acquires knowledge and skills appropriate to the neonatal specialty and practice setting.

Additional Measurement Criteria for the Advanced Practice Registered Nurse:

The advanced practice registered nurse uses current healthcare research findings and other evidence to expand clinical knowledge, enhance role performance, and increase knowledge of professional issues.

STANDARD 9. PROFESSIONAL PRACTICE EVALUATION

The neonatal nurse evaluates one's own nursing practice in relation to professional practice standards and guidelines, relevant statutes, rules, and regulations.

Measurement Criteria:

The neonatal nurse's practice conforms with current practice standards, guidelines, statutes, rules, and regulations.

The neonatal nurse:

1. Engages in performance appraisal on a regular basis, identifying areas of strengths as well as areas for professional development.

2. Seeks constructive feedback on an ongoing basis for the purpose of professional development.

3. Takes action to achieve professional goals identified during the performance appraisal process.

4. Participates in peer review as appropriate.

5. Demonstrates knowledge of current professional practice standards, laws, and regulations in their own individual practice.

Additional Measurement Criteria for the Advanced Practice Registered Nurse:

The advanced practice registered nurse engages in a formal process seeking feedback regarding one's own practice from peers, professional colleagues, and others.

STANDARD 10. COLLEGIALITY

The neonatal nurse interacts with, and contributes to the professional development of, peers, other healthcare providers, and team members as colleagues.

Measurement Criteria:

The neonatal nurse:

1. Shares knowledge and skills with colleagues.

2. Provides peers with constructive feedback regarding neonatal care and practice.

3. Interacts with colleagues to enhance one's own professional neonatal nursing practice.

4. Contributes to an environment that is conducive to the clinical education of nursing students, other healthcare trainees, and other employees, as appropriate.

5. Contributes to a supportive and healthy work environment.

Additional Measurement Criteria for the Advanced Practice Registered Nurse:

The advanced practice registered nurse:

• Models expert practice to interdisciplinary team members and healthcare consumers.

• Mentors other nurses and colleagues as appropriate.

• Participates with interdisciplinary teams that contribute to role development and advanced nursing practice and health care.

STANDARD 11. COLLABORATION

The neonatal nurse collaborates with the family or caregiver and others in the conduct of nursing practice.

Measurement Criteria:

The neonatal nurse:

1. Communicates with the family and other healthcare providers regarding neonatal care and nursing's role in the provision of care.

2. Collaborates with the family and other healthcare providers in the formulation of overall goals and the plan of care, and in healthcare decisions related to the care and the delivery of services.

3. Consults with other healthcare providers for neonatal care, as needed.

4. Initiates referrals, including provisions for continuity of care, as needed.

Additional Measurement Criteria for the Advanced Practice Registered Nurse:

The advanced practice registered nurse:

• Partners with other disciplines to enhance infant care through interdisciplinary activities such as education, consultation, management, technological development, or research opportunities.

• Facilitates an interdisciplinary process with other members of the healthcare team.

• Documents plan of care communications, rationales for plan of care changes, and collaborative discussions to improve infant care.

STANDARD 12. ETHICS

The neonatal nurse's decisions and actions on behalf of infants and their families or caregivers in all areas of practice are determined in an ethical manner.

Measurement Criteria:

The neonatal nurse:

1. Ensures that their practice is guided by *Nursing's Social Policy Statement, 2nd Edition* (ANA 2003) and *Code of Ethics for Nurses with Interpretive Statements* (ANA, 2001).

2. Maintains patient and family confidentiality within legal and regulatory parameters.

3. Acts as a patient advocate and assists the family in developing skills to become advocates for their child.

4. Delivers care in a nonjudgmental and nondiscriminatory manner that is sensitive to patient diversity.

5. Delivers care in a manner that preserves patient and family autonomy, dignity, and rights from first encounter through end-of-life care.

6. Utilizes available resources in formulating ethical decisions.

Additional Measurement Criteria for the Advanced Practice Registered Nurse:

The advanced practice registered nurse:

• Informs the family, caregiver, or other decisionmaker of the risks, benefits, and outcomes of healthcare regimens.

• Participates in multidisciplinary teams that evaluate ethical risks, benefits, and outcomes.

STANDARD 13. RESEARCH

The neonatal nurse integrates research findings into practice.

Measurement Criteria:

The neonatal nurse:

1. Utilizes the best available evidence (ideally scientific research findings) to develop the plan of care and interventions and guide practice decisions.

2. Participates in research activities at various levels appropriate to the nurse's education, experience, and position. These may include the following:

    • Identification of clinical problems pertinent to neonatal nursing care.

    • Participation in all aspects of the research process, as appropriate, including data collection.

    • Participation in unit, organizational, community, or global research activities.

    • Dissemination of research information and findings with peers and others.

    • Conducting research.

    • Critiquing of research for application to neonatal practice.

    • Use of research findings in the development of policies, procedures, and practice guidelines for neonatal care.

    • Use of research findings to advance the state of nursing science in the care of neonatal patients and families.

Additional Measurement Criteria for the Advanced Practice Registered Nurse:

The advanced practice registered nurse:

• Contributes to nursing knowledge by conducting or synthesizing research that discovers, examines and evaluates knowledge, theories, criteria, and creative approaches to improve healthcare practice.

• Formally disseminates research findings through activities such as presentations, publications, consultation, and journal clubs.

STANDARD 14. RESOURCE UTILIZATION

The neonatal nurse considers factors related to safety, effectiveness, cost, and impact on practice in the planning and delivering of nursing services.

Measurement Criteria:

The neonatal nurse:

1. Evaluates factors such as patient safety, effectiveness, availability, and cost when choosing among practice options having the same expected patient outcome.

2. Assists the family in identifying and securing necessary resources and services to address healthcare needs.

3. Assigns or delegates tasks as defined by the state Nurse Practice Acts and in accordance with the designated caregiver's knowledge, experience, and skills.

4. Assigns or delegates tasks based on the needs and condition of the infant, the potential for harm, the stability of the infant's condition, the complexity of the care, and the predictability of the outcome.

5. Assists the family or caregivers in becoming informed consumers with regard to risks, benefits, and cost of treatment and care.

Additional Measurement Criteria for the Advanced Practice Registered Nurse:

The advanced practice registered nurse:

- Utilizes organizational and community resources to formulate a multidisciplinary plan of care.

- Develops innovative solutions for infant care problems that address effective resource utilization and maintenance of quality.

- Develops evaluation strategies to demonstrate cost effectiveness, cost benefit, and efficiency factors associated with neonatal nursing practice.

The neonatal nurse provides leadership in the professional practice setting and the profession.

Measurement Criteria:

The neonatal nurse:

1. Engages in teamwork as a team player and a team builder.

2. Works to create and maintain healthy environments in local, regional, national, or international communities.

3. Displays the ability to define a clear vision, the associated goals, and a plan to implement and measure progress.

4. Demonstrates a commitment to continuous, lifelong learning for self and others.

5. Teaches others to succeed by mentoring and other strategies.

6. Exhibits creativity and flexibility through times of change.

7. Demonstrates energy, excitement, and a passion for quality work.

8. Willingly accepts mistakes by self and others, thereby creating a culture in which risk-taking is not only accepted, but expected.

9. Inspires loyalty through valuing of people as the most precious asset in an organization.

10. Directs the coordination of care across settings and among caregivers, including supervision of licensed and unlicensed personnel in any assigned or delegated tasks.

11. Serves in key roles in the work setting by participating on committees, councils, and administrative teams.

12. Promotes advancement of the profession through participation in professional organizations.

Continued ▸

Additional Measurement Criteria for the Advanced Practice Registered Nurse:

The advanced practice registered nurse:

- Works to influence policymaking bodies to improve infant care.

- Provides direction to enhance the effectiveness of the healthcare team.

- Initiates and revises protocols or guidelines to reflect evidence-based practice, to reflect accepted changes in care management, or to address emerging problems.

- Promotes communication and the advancement of the profession through writing, publishing, and presentations for professional or lay audiences.

- Designs innovations to effect change in practice and to improve health outcomes.

GLOSSARY

Assessment. A systematic data collection process used by the nurse, through interaction with the infant and family, significant others, and healthcare providers, to collect and analyze information regarding the health needs of the infant and family. Information collected may be related to the physiological, psychosocial, sociocultural, spiritual, environmental, educational, developmental, and discharge-planning needs of the infant and family. These data can be collected through observation, physical examination, medical record review, interviews, and discussion with family members, as well as perinatal, neonatal, and other healthcare providers, as appropriate.

Collaboration. Planning, implementing, and evaluating care, with consideration given to each discipline and the family's unique contribution to the care. Similar to collegiality, in that both require teamwork to achieve the desired care outcome.

Collegiality. A work ethic that involves working as a team in a professional and equal manner to achieve the expected care outcome.

Diagnosis. A clinical judgment made by a nurse regarding the infant or family responses to actual or potential health conditions or needs. Diagnoses provide the basis for determining a plan of care that will achieve expected outcomes.

Education. The degree to which the nurse keeps academically current in the neonatal nursing specialty.

Environment. The conditions, circumstances, and influences surrounding and affecting the infant and family, including the physical and caregiving environments. The physical environment refers to conditions such as lighting and noise levels and temperature fluctuations within an ambient space. The caregiving environment refers to the manner in which interventions are administered, the way the infant and family are handled, and the use of equipment when administering care (Gottfried, 1985).

Evaluation. The determination of the infant and family's progress toward the attainment of expected outcomes and the effectiveness of the nursing care delivered by the professional nurse; the final step in the nursing process.

Expected outcomes. Goals achieved as a result of care that can be objectively measured.

Family. Family of origin, significant others, or caregivers.

Guidelines. Recommended courses of action in various clinical situations or for specific client conditions or populations. Guidelines provide linkages among nursing diagnoses, interventions, and outcome. They also describe alternatives available to each patient and provide a basis for the evaluation of care and allocation of resources. Guidelines are recommendations for practice with supportive evidence from the literature.

Implementation. Activities used by the nurse to carry out the plan of care, including psychomotor skills, interviews, and coordination and delegation of care activities.

Infant. A baby in the first year of life.

Kangaroo care. The practice of resting an infant on a parent's bare chest to promote parent–infant bonding in babies requiring special care. Other benefits include earlier discharge from hospital, easier breast-feeding, and mutual comfort.

Neonate, Newborn. An infant 28 days of age or younger.

Performance appraisal. Measurement of the cognitive and behavioral aspects of the neonatal nurse's role.

Performance standards. Broad statements of professional nursing expectations. They include competencies and accountabilities for the professional nurse. They reflect criteria that are measurable.

Planning. Documenting the care to be delivered to the infant and family to attain the expected outcomes.

Quality of care. The degree to which the care rendered reflects the expected minimum level of care and the achievement of expected care outcomes, according to defined professional and consumer expectations.

Research. The systematic study of care practices or professional performance. Research yields evidence to support interventions.

Resource utilization. Awareness of the supports available and necessary for care, as well as use of those supports in a responsible manner to achieve quality of care.

Standards. Broad statements that address the basic scope of professional nursing practice. They identify minimum acceptable care practices for the professional nurse who cares for specific populations of patients. These standards are population-based and not setting-specific.

REFERENCES

American Nurses Association. (2001). *Code of ethics for nurses with interpretive statements.* Washington, DC: American Nurses Publishing. (See also http://www.nursingworld.org/ethics/ecode.htm)

American Nurses Association. (2003). *Nursing's social policy statement, 2nd edition.* Washington, DC: nursesbooks.org.

American Nurses Association (2004). *Nursing: Scope and standards of practice.* Washington, DC: nursesbooks.org.

Bagwell et al. (2003) Regionalization in today's healthcare delivery system. In

Kenner, C. & Wright Lott, J., editors, *Comprehensive neonatal nursing, 3rd Edition.* St. Louis, MO: Mosby.

Harrigan, R.C. & Perez, D.J. (2003). Neonatal nursing in the new healthcare delivery environment. In Kenner, C. & Wright Lott, J., editors. *Comprehensive neonatal nursing, 3rd Edition.* St. Louis, MO: Mosby.

Human Genome Project. (2004). www.ornl.gov/sci/technsource/Human_Genome/home.shtml

Joint Commission on Accreditation of Healthcare Organizations. (2003). *Comprehensive accreditation manual for hospitals.* Oakbrook Terrace, IL: JCAHO.

National Association of Neonatal Nurses. (1999a). *Advanced practice neonatal nurse role* (No. 3000). Glenview, IL: NANN.

National Association of Neonatal Nurses. (1999b). *Cultural competence* (No. 3037). Glenview, IL: NANN.

National Association of Neonatal Nurses. (1999c). *Transport of neonates across state lines* (No. 3020). Glenview, IL: NANN.

Stevens, K.R. (2003). Evidence-based neonatal nursing practice. In Kenner, C. & Wright Lott, J., editors. *Comprehensive neonatal nursing, 3rd Edition.* St. Louis, MO: Mosby.

(Note: All URLs were confirmed active as of March 30, 2004.)

Bibliography

American Academy of Pediatrics. (2000). *Policy statement prevention and management of pain stress in the neonate* (RE9945). Elk Grove Village, IL: AAP.

American Academy of Pediatrics and American College of Obstetricians and Gynecologists. (2002). *Guidelines for perinatal care, 5th Ed.* Elk Grove Village, IL: AAP.

American Nurses Association. (2001). Press release: ANA House of Delegates Passes Revised Code of Ethics. Washington, DC: ANA.

American Nurses Association (2002). *Scope and standards of neuroscience nursing practice.* Washington, DC: American Nurses Publishing.

Association of Women's Health, Obstetric, and Neonatal Nurses. (1997). *Guidelines of neonatal nursing: Orientation and development for Registered and Advanced Practice Nurses in basic and intensive care settings.* Washington, DC: AWHONN.

Association of Women's Health, Obstetric, and Neonatal Nurses. (1998). *Standards and guidelines for professional nursing practice in the care of women and newborns, 5th Ed.* Washington, DC: AWHONN.

Carrera, J. M., Chervenak, F. A., and Kurjak, A. (2003). *Controversies in perinatal medicine: The fetus as a patient.* Boca Raton, FL: CRC Press-Parthenon Publishers. (This book was developed from the 2003 proceedings in Barcelona, Spain of the 19th International Congress of the Society of the Fetus as Patient.)

Carter, B.S. (2001). *Ethical issues in neonatal care.* www.emedicine.com

Gottfried, A.W. (1985). Environment of newborn in special care units. In Gottfried, A.W.& Gaiter, J.L. eds. *Infant stress under intensive care.* Baltimore: University Park Press.

National Association of Neonatal Nurses. (1999). *NICU nurse involvement in ethical decisions (Treatment of critically ill newborns).* (No. 3015). Glenview, IL: NANN.

National Association of Neonatal Nurses. (1999). *Standards of care for neonatal nursing practice.* Glenview, IL: NANN.

National Association of Neonatal Nurses. (2003). *FAQs.* www.nann.org

National Association of Neonatal Nurses. (2003). *History.* www.nann.org

Sheeran, Brophy MS. (2001). Nurse advocacy in the neonatal unit: Putting theory into practice. *Journal of Neonatal Nursing*, 7(1) 10–11.

Smington, A. & Pinelli, J. (2003). *Developmental care for promoting development and preventing morbidity in preterm infants*. Cochrane Library *(Cochrane Review)*.

World Health Organization. (2004). *Child and adolescent health and development: Prevention and care of Illness: Neonates and infants*. Geneva: WHO. http://www.who.int/child-adolescent-health/

(Note: All URLs were confirmed active as of March 30, 2004.)

APPENDIX A
Provisions of the ANA Code of Ethics for Nurses

1. The nurse, in all professional relationships, practices with compassion and respect for the inherent dignity, worth and uniqueness of every individual, unrestricted by considerations of social or economic status, personal attributes, or the nature of health problems.

2. The nurse's primary commitment is to the patient, whether an individual, family, group, or community.

3. The nurse promotes, advocates for, and strives to protect the health, safety, and rights of the patient.

4. The nurse is responsible and accountable for individual nursing practice and determines the appropriate delegation of tasks consistent with the nurse's obligation to provide optimum patient care.

5. The nurse owes the same duties to self as to others, including the responsibility to preserve integrity and safety, to maintain competence, and to continue personal and professional growth.

6. The nurse participates in establishing, maintaining, and improving healthcare environments and conditions of employment conducive to the provision of quality health care and consistent with the values of the profession through individual and collective action.

7. The nurse participates in the advancement of the profession through contributions to practice, education, administration, and knowledge development.

8. The nurse collaborates with other health professionals and the public in promoting community, national, and international efforts to meet health needs.

9. The profession of nursing, as represented by associations and their members, is responsible for articulating nursing values, for maintaining the integrity of the profession and its practice, and for shaping social policy.

Source: American Nurses Association (2001).*Code of Ethics for Nurses with Interpretive Statements.* Washington, D.C.: American Nurses Publishing.

INDEX

Collegiality
assumptions regarding, *ix*
defined, 29
leadership and, 27
professional practice evaluation
and, 21
research and, 25
standard of professional
performance, 22
Communication
in framework of neonatal
nursing, 1
home care and, 6
leadership and, 27
research and, 25
See also Collaboration;
Consultation
Community health
coordination of care and, 14
discharge planning and, 2
implementation and, 13
research and, 25
resource utilization and, 26
Competence assessment. *See*
Certification and credentialing
Confidentiality
ethics and, 24
See also Ethics
Consultation
collaboration and, 23
leadership and, 27
research and, 25
standard of practice, 16
Continuity of care
collaboration and, 23
coordination of care and, 14
outcome identification and, 11
planning and, 12
Coordination of care, *x*
environment and, 2
health promotion and, 2
implementation and, 30

leadership and, 27
standard of practice, 14
See also Interdisciplinary health
care
Coping, 1
Cost control
insurance and, 7
prescriptive authority and, 16
resource utilization and, 26
Cost-effectiveness. *See* Cost control
Credentialing. *See* Certification and
credentialing
Criteria for standards, *x–xi*, 9–28
assessment, 9
collaboration, 23
collegiality, 22
consultation, 16
coordination of care, 14
diagnosis, 10
education, 20
ethics, 24
evaluation, 17
health teaching and health
promotion, 15
implementation, 13–16
leadership, 27–28
outcome identification, 11
planning, 12
prescriptive authority and
treatment, 16
professional practice evaluation,
21
quality of practice, 19–20
research, 25
resource utilization, 26
Critical thinking, analysis, and
synthesis
assessment and, 9
consultation and, 16
coordination of care and, 14
diagnosis and, 10
education and, 20

ethics and, 2
evaluation and, 17
health promotion and, 15
quality of practice and, 19
research and, 25
Cultural competence
assumptions regarding, *ix*
ethics and, 24
in framework of neonatal
nursing, 2
health promotion and, 15
outcome identification and, 11
planning and, 12
See also Spiritual care

D
Data collection
assessment and, 9, 29
diagnosis and, 10
planning and, 12
quality of practice and, 19
research and, 25
Delivery room, 3, 4, 5, 6
Decision-making
collaboration and, 23
consultation and, 16
ethics and, 2, 6
planning and, 12
research and, 25
Developmental care, 1
diagnosis and, 10
family and, 3
in framework of neonatal
nursing, 2
health promotion and, 15
implementation and, 13
planning and, 12
Diagnosis
assessment and, 9
defined, 29
differential, 10
evaluation and, 17

guidelines and, 30
outcome identification and, 11
planning and, 12
prescriptive authority and, 16
quality of practice and,
standard of practice, 10
Discharge planning
assessment and, 29
diagnosis and, 10
in framework of neonatal
nursing, 2
kangaroo care and, 30
Level II care and, 4
trends, 6
Documentation
assessment and, 9
collaboration and, 23
coordination of care and, 14
diagnosis and, 10
evaluation and, 17
health promotion and, 15
implementation and, 13
planning and, 12, 30

E
Economic issues. *See* Cost control
Education of families, 1
assumptions regarding, *ix*
diagnosis and, 10
ethics and, 24
health promotion and, 15
planning and, 12
prescriptive authority and, 16
resource utilization and, 26
See also Family; Health teaching
and health promotion; Patient
Education of neonatal nurses, 5
àssumptions regarding, *ix*
collaboration and, 23
collegiality and, 22
defined, 29
leadership and, 27

neonatal clinical nurse specialist
and, 5
neonatal nurse practitioner and, 5
research and, 25
standard of professional
performance, 20
See also Mentoring; Professional
development
Environment
collegiality and, 22
coordination of care and, 14
defined, 29
diagnosis and, 10
in framework of neonatal
nursing, 2
implementation and, 13
quality of practice and, 19
See also Practice environment
Ethics
assumptions regarding, *ix*
codes, *vii*, 24
in framework of neonatal
nursing, 2
standard of professional
performance, 24
trends, 6
See also Laws, statutes, and
regulations
Evaluation
collaboration and, 29
defined, 29
guidelines and, 30
health promotion and, 2, 15
leadership and, 27
planning and, 12
prescriptive authority and, 16
quality of practice and, 19
standard of practice, 17
Evidence-based practice
assumptions regarding, *ix*
consultation and, 16

discharge planning and, 2
guidelines and, 30
leadership and, 27
neonatal clinical nurse specialist
and, 5
outcome identification and, 11
prescriptive authority and, 16
quality of practice and, 19, 20
research and, 6, 25, 30
See also Research
Expected outcomes. *See* Outcomes

F
Family
advocacy, 4
assessment and, 9, 29
assumptions regarding, *ix*
bond with newborn, 1, 2
collaboration and, 5, 23
communication and, 1
consultation and, 16
coping, 1
defined, 30
diagnosis and, 10
discharge planning and, 4
ethics and, 2, 24
evaluation and, 17
health promotion and, 15
implementation and, 13
outcome identification and, 11
planning and, 12
prescriptive authority and, 16
resource utilization and, 26
See also Education of families;
Patient
Family-focused care
in framework of neonatal
nursing, 3
See also Family
Fetal surgery, 6
Financial issues. *See* Cost control

Framework of neonatal nursing
   practice, 1–3
      communication, 1
      culturally sensitive care, 2
      developmental care, 2
      discharge planning, 2
      ethical decision-making, 2
      environment, 2
      family-focused care, 3
      health promotion, 2
      quality assurance and research, 3
      spiritual care, 3

G

Gene therapy, 6
Generalist neonatal nursing
   assessment, 9
   collaboration, 23
   collegiality, 22
   consultation, 16
   coordination of care, 14
   diagnosis, 10
   education, 5, 20
   ethics, 24
   evaluation, 17
   health teaching and health
      promotion, 15
   implementation, 13–16
   leadership, 27
   outcome identification, 11
   planning, 12
   prescriptive authority and
      treatment, 16
   professional practice evaluation,
      21
   quality of practice, 19
   research, 25
   resource utilization, 26
   roles, 5
   See also Advanced practice
      neonatal nursing; Neonatal
      nursing

Guidelines
   defined, 30
   leadership and, 27, 28
   outcome identification and, 11
   professional practice evaluation
      and, 21
   quality of practice and, 19
   research and, 25
   trends, 6

H

Health teaching and health promotion
   evaluation and, 4
   in framework of neonatal
      nursing, 2
   leadership and, 27
   standard of practice, 15
   See also Education of families
Healthcare policy
   assumptions regarding, *ix*
   evaluation and, 17
   implementation and, 13
   leadership and, 28
   quality of practice and, 19, 20
   research and, 25
Healthcare providers
   assessment and, 9, 29
   assumptions regarding, *ix*
   collaboration and, 23
   collegiality and, 22
   communication and, 1
   diagnosis and, 10
   evaluation and, 17
   insurance and, 7
   leadership and, 27, 28
   outcome identification and, 11
   planning and, 12
   quality of practice and, 19
   transport care and, 4
   See also Collaboration;
      Coordination of care;
      Interdisciplinary healthcare

education and, 5
leadership and, 27
professional practice evaluation
and, 21
See also Education of neonatal
nurses
Mother, 3
See also Family
Multidisciplinary healthcare. *See*
Interdisciplinary health care

N
National Association of Neonatal
Nurses (NANN), *vii*
Neonatal Clinical Nurse
Specialist (NCNS), 5, 7
Neonatal intensive care unit (NICU),
vii, 4, 6
Neonatal Nurse Clinicians
Practitioners and Specialists, *vii*
Neonatal Nurse Practitioner (NNP), 5, 7
Neonatal Nurses Association, *vii*
Neonatal Nurses of Northern
California, *vii*
Neonatal nursing
advanced practice, 5
certification, 5
characteristics, 1–3
defined, 1
education, 5
environment 3–5
framework of practice, 1–3
generalist practice, 5
historical background, *vii*
practice environment, 3–5
professional development, 5, 6
qualifications, 5
research, 6
scope of practice, 1–7
shortage, 7
skills, 1
support of, 6

trends, 6–7
See also Advanced practice
neonatal nursing; Generalist
neonatal nursing
Neonatal nursing advanced level. *See*
Advanced practice neonatal nursing
Neonate (defined), 30
Newborn (defined), 30
Nursery, 7
practice setting, 3
Nursing care standards. *See*
Standards of practice
Nursing standards. *See* Standards of
practice; Standards of professional
performance
Nursing's Social Policy Statement, viii, 24

O
Outcome identification
standard of practice, 11
See also Outcomes
Outcomes
defined, 29
diagnosis and, 10
ethics and, 24
evaluation and, 4, 17
guidelines and, 30
implementation and, 13
planning and, 12
resource utilization and, 26
See also Outcome identification

P
Pain management, 1, 2, 9
Parents. *See* Family
Patient
advocacy, 4
assessment and, 9, 29
assumptions regarding, *ix*
diagnosis and, 10
ethics and, 24
evaluation and, 17

implementation and, 13
outcome identification and, 11
planning and, 12
prescriptive authority and, 16
resource utilization and, 26
See also Education of families;
Family
Performance appraisal (defined), 30
Performance standards (defined), 30
See also Standards
Pharmacologic agents. *See* Prescriptive
authority and treatment
Planning
collaboration and, 23, 29
consultation and, 16
defined, 30
diagnosis and, 10
discharge and, 6
evaluation and, 17
health promotion and, 2
implementation and, 13, 30
leadership and, 27
outcome identification and, 4, 11
research and, 25
resource utilization and, 26
standard of practice, 12
Policy. *See* Healthcare policy
Practice environment, 3–5
characteristics, 1–3
See also Environment
Practice settings, 3–4
delivery room, 3
Level I, 3
Level II, 4
Level III, 4
transport, 4
Practice standards. *See* Standards of
practice
Preceptors. *See* Mentoring
Premature Institute, *vii*

Premature newborns, 4, 7
Prescriptive authority and treatment
standard of practice, 16
Preventive care. *See* Health teaching
and health promotion
Privacy. *See* Confidentiality
Professional development, 5
collegiality and, 22
education and, 20
leadership and, 27, 28
professional practice evaluation
and, 21
research and, 6
See also Education of neonatal
nurses; Leadership
Professional performance. *See*
Standards of professional
performance
Professional practice evaluation
standard of professional
performance, 21

Q
Quality of practice
assumptions regarding, *ix*
defined, 30
in framework of neonatal
nursing, 3
neonatal clinical nurse specialist
and, 5
research and, 3
resource utilization and, 26
standard of professional
performance, 19–20

R
Recipient of care. *See* Patient
Recruitment and retention, 6, 7
leadership and, 27
See also Professional development

Referral
    collaboration and, 23
    prescriptive authority and, 16
Regulatory issues. *See* Laws, statutes,
    and regulations
Reimbursement, 7
Research
    in advanced practice, 5
    assumptions regarding, *ix*
    collaboration and, 23
    defined, 30
    education and, 20
    evidence-based practice and, 6
    in framework of neonatal
        nursing, 3
    future trends, 6
    planning and, 12
    quality of practice and, 3, 19, 20
    standard of professional
        performance, 25
    See also Evidence-based practice
Resource utilization
    assumptions regarding, *ix*
    defined, 30
    ethics and, 24
    health promotion and, 15
    implementation and, 13
    standard of professional
        performance, 26
Risk assessment
    ethics and, 24
    health promotion and, 15
    leadership and, 27
    prescriptive authority and, 16
    resource utilization and, 26
    See also High-risk neonates

S
Safety assurance
    collegiality and, 22
    health promotion and, 15
    implementation and, 13

quality of practice and,
    resource utilization and, 26
Scientific findings. *See* Evidence-
    based practice; Research
Scope of practice, 1–7
Scope and Standards of Practice Task
    Force, *vii*
Settings. *See* Practice settings
Significant others. *See* Family
Special care, 4
Spiritual care in neonatal nursing, 3
    nursing, 3
    See also Cultural competence
Staffing issues. *See* Recruitment and
    retention
Standards, *vii-viii*, 9–28
    defined, 30
    historical background, *vii*
    professional practice evaluation
        and, 21
    underlying assumptions, *ix*
    See also Standards of practice;
        Standards of professional
        performance
Standards of practice, *vii*, 9–17
    assessment, 9
    consultation, 16
    coordination of care, 14
    diagnosis, 10
    evaluation, 17
    health teaching and health
        promotion, 15
    implementation, 13–16
    outcome identification, 11
    planning, 12
    prescriptive authority and
treatment, 16
Standards of professional
    performance, *vii*, 19–28
    collaboration, 23
    collegiality, 22
    education, 20

ethics, 24
leadership, 27–28
professional practice evaluation,
    21
quality of practice, 19–20
research, 25
resource utilization, 26
Support of neonatal nursing, 6
Synthesis. *See* Critical thinking,
  analysis, and synthesis

T

Teaching. *See* Education of families;
  Education of neonatal nurses;
  Health teaching and health
  promotion
Teams and teamwork. *See*
  Collaboration; Interdisciplinary
  health care
Transitional care, 4
Transport care, 4
Trends in neonatal nursing, 6–7

ANA NURSING STANDARDS PACKAGE

The set—totaling over 1,000 pages—contains **the newly revised keystone publication of the set,** *Nursing: Scope and Standards of Practice,* **plus one each of the current volume for the 22 nursing specialty areas** listed below. Each volume delineates and discusses the scope, status, and prospects of that specialized practice along with its generalist competencies, any advanced practice competencies, and the evidence-based standards with measurement criteria for practice and professional performance.

Pub# *PKG*   *List $330/Member $260*

The ANA Standards Package contains:

NURSING: SCOPE AND STANDARDS OF PRACTICE, 2004/126 pp. (*NEW EDITION*)
   Provides the standards for clinical, non-clinical, and advanced practice; includes the 1973, 1981, 1991, and 1997 editions.
#04SSNP   **List $19.95/Member $16.95**

… plus 22 additional scope and standards of specialty practice*, all affordably priced at List $16.95/Member $13.45:
The latest additions to the set…

Nurse Administrators, 2004 (*NEW EDITION*)	#03SSNA	**Nursing Professional Development,** 2000	#NPD20
Addictions Nursing, 2004 (*NEW EDITION*)	#04SSAN	**Palliative & Hospice Nursing,** 2002	#HPN22
Neonatal Nursing, 2004 (*FIRST EDITION*)	#04SSNN	**Parish Nursing,** 1998	#9806ST
Vascular Nursing, 2004 (*FIRST EDITION*)	#04SSVN	**Pediatric Nursing,** 2003 (*NEW EDITION*)	#PNP23
… join		**Pediatric Oncology Nursing,** 2000	#PONP20
College Health Nursing, 1997	# ST1	**Psychiatric–Mental Health Nursing,** 2000	#PMH20
Correctional Facilities Nursing, 1995	#NP104	**Public Health Nursing,** 1999	#910PH
Developmental Disabilities		**School Nursing,** 2001	#SHNP21
and/or Mental Retardation, 1998	#9802ST		
Diabetes Nursing, 2ⁿᵈ Edition, 2003	#DNP23		
Forensic Nursing, 1997	#ST4		
Genetics Clinical Nursing, 1998	#9807ST		
Gerontological Nursing, 2ⁿᵈ Edition, 2001	#GNP21		
Home Health Nursing, 1999	#9905HH		
Neuroscience Nursing, 2002	#NNS22		
Nursing Informatics, 2001	#NIP21		

ANA STANDARDS STANDING ORDER PLAN
Great plan for university, hospital, and medical center libraries! Get the newest Standards as soon as they are published. We'll send the book along with an invoice. Plus, you'll save 10% off list price.
(*ANA members receive an additional 20% savings.*)
For details, or to enroll, call (800) 637-0323.

(* Titles may be ordered separately.)

ORDER FORM

Title	Price	Qty	Total
Nursing Standards Package #PKG			
	Shipping & Handling		
TOTAL			

Shipping and Handling	U.S.	Outside U.S.
Up to $25	$4	$8
25.01–$50	$6	$12
$50.01–$100	$8	$16
$100.01–$200	$14	$24
$200.01–$300	$12	$32
$300.01⁺	7% of total	15% of total

Shipping: 7–10 days for domestic deliveries. 7–30 business days for international deliveries. Items cannot be delivered to a P.O. box. All orders must include shipping and handling charges.

Payment: (payment in U.S. dollars required)
[   ] Check enclosed (made payable to *American Nurses Association*)
Charge my [   ] VISA   [   ] MasterCard

Card # _____ **Exp Date** _____

Signature _____

Phone # _____ **CMA#** _____ **

** Your CMA I.D. number must be provided to receive member discount.
   20% discount off list price on orders of 20+ copies of the same title.

Ship to:
Name _____

Organization _____

Address _____

City/State/Zip _____

Phone # _____ **Fax #** _____

HOW TO ORDER